# IN A RISING WIND

## A Personal Journey
## Through Dyslexia

## Paul C. Ziminsky

UNIVERSITY
PRESS OF
AMERICA

Lanham • New York • London

Copyright © 1993 by
**University Press of America®, Inc.**
4720 Boston Way
Lanham, Maryland 20706

3 Henrietta Street
London WC2E 8LU England

**Library of Congress Cataloging-in-Publication Data**

Ziminsky, Paul C.
In a rising wind : a personal journey through dyslexia /
by Paul C. Ziminsky.
p.    cm.
1. Dyslexic children—Education.   2. Dyslexia.
3. Ziminsky, Paul C.   4. Dyslexics—Biography.   I. Title.
LC4708.Z56    1993      371.91'44—dc20      92–42527  CIP

ISBN 0–8191–9049–7 (pbk. : alk. paper)

# *Dedication*

*This paper is dedicated to my best friend, me, in the hope that I may continue to stand by my own side and believe in myself in order to live a full life and be there for others.*

# *Acknowledgments*

I would like to thank Dr. Fournier, William Flavin, Peter Hainer, Alan Hunter, Dr. Steinburg, Dr. Webb and all professors at Curry College for the support and guidance they have given me. Also, I acknowledge my friends for their continued support in helping me accomplish my goals. I am grateful to Dr. Warners and all of the people involved with the Honors Program. I thank my advisor Joe Arsenault for caring, and the incredible support and understanding that he provided, from day one. If not for Joe the story never would have been started. Finally, I am grateful to my main mentor Ned Bradford, for without his patience, understanding and friendship this story would never have been finished.

# *Preface*

I have written a story on the problem of growing up with a disability in our society to serve as an allegory for anyone with a difference who must live in a society that cannot handle differences well.

In the socialization process, the goal is conformity. In many cases the socialization process drives people who are learning disabled towards low self- esteem and eventual learned helplessness, because their learning differences make it difficult for them to fit in.

This state of learned helplessness is important to understand in order to assist people with learning disabilities break the pattern. When we understand the phenomena we can change. And parents and teachers can avoid setting students up to become "learned helpless."

It was clear to me that I have a degree of learned helplessness. And once this realization was made I found I had a responsibility to myself to find out more and do whatever I could to get back to reality so that I could live a positive life, instead of a self defeating life.

Persistence, Patience, Being Nice To Myself is what it was all about.

Here is my story...................

# *Chapter 1*

## WHAT THE HELL WAS GOING ON

Back in seventh grade at St. Francis is when I began getting sick of it. They were all the same, every paper I ever wrote. Why would I think that this time it would be different? I do not know, maybe it was just wishful thinking.

I had tried. In fact I spent hours on the paper. I knew the subject matter...I was actually excited about it.

"Paul, I can see that you have a good grasp of the subject, but this paper is very poorly written. You have got to spend more time on your work. You cannot expect to pass without putting some effort into your work. But I will pass you anyway."

"But I will pass you anyway" brought on the idea that when I did pass, someone was just doing me a favor. A favor that can cripple. Taking success away from a child is taking away his or her existence.

In big, deep, dark, crimson, there it would be, along with a D. And of course everything else that went along with it.

# *Chapter 2*

## TIRED OF KNOWINGLY FURTHER COMPLICATING MY LIFE WITH LEARNED HELPLESSNESS

I was back at college after vowing never to return. I didn't need it. School was too painful.

My school career had been a failure, but I knew I was missing something. I was unsure of what it was and somehow I thought that I should give school and myself another chance. It took weeks of debating within; then I decided to go for it.

Stepping back into a classroom really brought back the fears of being inadequate to the surface. My body tensed and my mind would race as all the old failure fears arose. Was I setting myself up again to fail?

Having lunch with a few friends at Curry College, I noticed in them some of the same feelings that I felt way back when the poor grades started rolling in.

We were saying, mostly in roundabout ways:

"Why don't I ever finish a task?"

"Why am I such a bad student?"

"Why do I always wait to the last minute to get at a task when I know doing so makes success close to impossible?"

"Why am I such a fool?"

"Why do I think, if I cannot do it perfectly the first time that I should not try at all, when deep down inside I know that to do things well takes practice, persistence and patience?"

"Why can I not accept success?"

"Why do I always find reasons to say that I was lucky to succeed, or that any fool could do it?"

Over and over again these students and I would pound at ourselves. I tried to tell them that it was okay. I tried to tell them that they were awesome people and to just keep at it, that things would come around. Everything would be all right.

I soon realized that I was kidding myself. I knew the power of the helpless feeling. When I got honest with myself, I was able to see that the helpless feeling still had a strong hold on me.

But what could I do about it? I asked myself.

Can anything be done?

I majored in psychology hoping to find some answers. And through my studies I learned one of the most basic facts, which is that we need to see what we are dealing with or it is impossible to change. I saw that parent and teacher expectations could mean everything. We need to believe students can do it. In many cases because of the needs of the system to have everybody fit in to certain categories, the expectation for success is not there at all. What needs to be worked on may be something not in the other people, but in ourselves, where we can actually get something done. It was time to take a look within, try to put the past as far behind as I could and take a look at the realities of the day.

Then I found that after years of knocking oneself a thing called helplessness emerges. Learned helplessness refers to the perception of being helpless to control events. Seligman coined the term in 1975, when trying to understand adult depression and its effects. He observed that dogs subjected to unavoidable shocks in the laboratory eventually stopped producing coping responses. Even when free to escape they learned not to try. This scared the hell out of me.

Similarities between the experimentally induced "helpless" behavior and the behavior of depressed people led him to postulate that with learned helplessness, a person comes to expect that the outcomes of events are independent of his or her personal response. Thus, the person just stops trying, which in turn stops or slows down further learning -- a potentially devastating cycle. Although learned helplessness began as an explanation for adult depression, researchers have found it to be a useful construct for understanding many of the problems seen in children with learning problems.

Learning about child development, I saw that one's life script is made up at an incredibly early age. Some children's scripts are made up by eight years old. The script can be changed but if it has been reinforced for years, it can be difficult.

This is going to be a job, I thought. My life script was a negative one and it had been reinforced for a long time. Knowing that, I knew that there would be a strong force within, setting me up to fail. But I started this "recovery thing." I could see hope, really see it for what seemed like the first time in my life. I continued to learn more and tried to remember that I had set out to give myself another chance.

But the depth and the power of the life script and the learned helpless kid dying to fit in was awesome. I did not know exactly what I was going to do; I did not fully believe that I could change.

I had been at Curry for a year and a half. I was doing well building up positive experiences and successes, trying desperately to accept them. But the comfortable negative was always near.

A week later, I was asked if I would want to join the Honors Program.

Are you kidding? No way, I said to myself.

I said. "What will that mean?"

"It will mean that you will have the opportunity to work on a project of your own choosing for the next year and a half. You will not be totally on your own. There will be support throughout."

It all sounded pretty good, and pretty scary at the same time. But I would have a structured chance to put much of what I had learned, and what I knew I needed to learn, into some sort of package for myself and possibly for others. I knew I had to stay aware of the power of learned helplessness in order to keep moving away from the negative. It was not clear which way I was going to turn.

I could not avoid seeing repeats of the conversation I had at lunch with my buddies. The problem is real. This helplessness stuff, this setting oneself up for failure. I see it happening all over. I see it in me. It has got to stop. Maybe I can do it. I have to take responsibility. I have to take a chance.

### The Fog

The fog is thick.
Though the sun burns through.
Behind the tree is a cold dark building.
The traffic is getting louder in the street.
The children are playing in the school yard.
Behind the school is a windowless prison.

I needed to study learned helplessness, lack of motivation and low self-esteem further. I wanted to put it together in my head so that I could move on. But only I knew this. When I spoke, it was of others; not me. I did not have a problem. Again, I knew that I would have the ingrained urge to run and that I could easily be running again. I was so damn used to the running. So I joined the Honors Program and my topic would be my problem. Still, I would not have to admit anything and to run would be harder.

Before long, my project changed from showing that learned helplessness went hand in hand with differences that make it difficult to do school-related tasks, through a story; to the problem of learned helplessness and that it could easily overpower the problem of the learning differences and cause havoc in one's life; to a story about animals with learned helplessness, struggling and straggling to survive; to a story about me who has learned helplessness and how working at recovery one day at a time is vital, to avoid the straggle.

I set myself up on the third floor of an old Victorian, way up high with the great pines and oaks towering high outside my window. I have my plants, that have been with me since I came back to college three years ago, my music, my pictures, and a computer that just might help me get the story out.

Now it was really time to look back and within.


**PARENTCHILD     CHILDPARENT**

Frightening looking in,
Afraid to speak out.
Time to begin.
There is no doubt.
Where to begin?
The child knows.
The parent fears,
What he doesn't know.

All the child wants,
Is to be.
All the parent wants,
Is to be the child.


*It was a spring-like day towards the end of winter, oddly warm, bright and sunny. The younger trees were having a hard time. They were wondering if the bright, warm day was for real? Was spring here? Or was winter just taking a break?*

*The tree, thickest with age, said, "It is time for us to start letting our sap flow and get ready to grow again. I have been around for years and this is it. Spring is here to stay."*

*A young tree said, "Are you sure? Is it really that time again so soon?"*

*"See that stump over there?" the older tree said.*

*"Yes," said the small tree with shallow roots.*

*"Well, that was my father. He lived for two hundred years and he never steered me wrong."*

*Most of the trees that were close enough to hear the wise old tree, some of the smaller trees and bushes, went right along, no more questions asked. They figured that the thick tree knew the system pretty well. He had his own experience and the experience of even thicker trees and stumps from the past to back him up.*

*Who knows, they might have even made up the system, thought some of the younger trees as they began to sprout.*

*Just as they all started to bud, another towering tree spoke. "I have been growing in this forest for a long time and I think that there are many ways to grow. You do not have to follow along with my friend here who helps block the damaging winds from my branches. Most of the trees and grasses in this part of the forest have been following systems; but on very still summer nights I have heard others talk of living for a thousand years and more. It seems that they believe in doing whatever it is that comes naturally.''*

*''Well...........????? It's easier to fit in, to go along with the elders of the forest that we can see,'' said a few bushes.*

*''It may be easier for some. For others it could be an incredible waste of precious energy. Anyway, which ever way you choose good luck! Keep on growing; try and listen to your roots. As long as you know you have a choice. I'm going to save my strength for another day. See you later.''*

*''See ya.''*

*''Yes, thanks for the input.''*

*Some thought the second older tree was an idiot. Some thought the first tree was. Some concentrated on themselves, trying to hear what their own roots were saying. They were not sure what natural meant. They saved their decision for later.*

*The forest became speckled with green. Life went on. The warm spell lasted for a few days. Some of the trees were so indecisive that they wasted more energy than it would take to fully bloom. It was difficult standing in the uncertainty, unsure of what was to come.*

*With a burst of bitter cold, winter came back; the ground froze solid; it crackled and the branches did too. All the trees were forced to go back to sleep. The forest was quiet.*

*When spring slowly arrived, most trees turned green and shot towards the sun, except for the few who had spent the last of their energy when tricked by the early thaw. Others grew stronger from the adversity. Some went along growing strong, slowly and well, listening quietly to their roots, accepting the uncertainty.*

I leaned back from my computer looking at the trees, and thought. What the hell is this? What am I doing? I can't write. Who am I kidding? I read my first book three years ago and now I think I can write one of my own. Who am I kidding? This is stupid.

Hold on, Paul. You know what you are up against. All right, I will go over it briefly and see if that helps.

Happiness grows out of looking at things in a different light so that the good outweighs the bad. You know that, Paul, so take a deep breath and look at the good.

It is okay to look back; it is possible to make some new decisions about what you can and cannot do. Give yourself that chance.

You have to take responsibility, Paul. Take a chance. You do not have to have an answer.

What about that inner push or pull toward peace and happiness? You are all right. Go with it, let it happen.

Okay, what is it? What happened? I thought, as I continued to gaze at the beauty outside my window. I have a choice. It is up to me. All right, let's see.

# *Chapter 3*

## TEACHERS TAUGHT BY TEACHERS

My first day in kindergarten was a big day. It was supposed to be fun and fun it was. We had big red building blocks, tons of crayons, paper and glue. We did fun things; we made pictures for our parents, ran around some, had a snack time, a nap time, then went home for lunch. It was simple. It was easy. It was nice being happy and carefree. Everything was in tune, balanced, effortless. Without a worry in the world, I would walk home from the bus stop, singing and kicking stones on the dirt road that led to my house, thinking of the fluffanutter sandwich and chocolate milk waiting for me.

As I grew and moved from room to room, first grade to second, the simplicity left. All the rooms were pretty much the same, though. They were square and colorless. The desks were lined in neat rows with a bigger desk (front and center) for the teacher.

I noticed quickly that I could not read like the other kids. At first it was no big deal. I learned how to hide in the back of the class. But later, it was necessary to produce things for the teacher, written things. I could hide no longer. They had me.

What is wrong with me? I thought. It was scary and humiliating at times.

Humiliation; what was that?

I knew it hurt.

I knew it scared me.

But why?

Why?

What was wrong with me?

Is this the way it's going to be?

I was in penmanship class one day, when the witch, Sister Richard, asked me to come up to her desk.

"Yes," I said in a frightened voice.

"What is this letter?" she said, with her eyes peering at me like a person does when they know they have you up against a wall.

I scoped her desk, looking for something, anything to help me out of the jam. What was it that I needed? It was one of those vowel things. But which one was it?

I had developed a talent in writing so that my vowels all looked alike. It made it a little easier to fool the teachers. Ambiguity was safe. No one could call me to task. Everything was up in the air.

"What do you think it is, sister?"

"It looks like it is an 'o' but it should be an 'a'... it could also be an 'e', well I guess it could be an 'a'."

"Well, it is an 'a', Sister."

"You have got to start trying to write more clearly, Paul."

"Yes, Sister, I will try to be more careful with my writing." If I could not find what I needed I would get her to answer her own question. Then I would go on my way, to the back of the class, hoping to go unseen for the rest of the day. I felt like an alien in a strangely twisted place where the air was slowly choking the life from me. And on the other hand, I felt there was something wrong with me. I must not be good enough. Many days, hiding would work. But all too often it would not. I was scared almost all the time now. My life had become miserable so fast. It was hard to believe. Everyone was wondering what was happening to the happy-go-lucky me. I was, too. The only answer I came up with was that it was me. I did not fit in. Something was wrong with me. "I am not good enough" became the tape playing in my head.

Later that year, one rainy school day while waiting for the dreaded school bus, the fear ran through my veins, my whole body tensed up, ready to jump, kill or be killed. It hurt to be at school. It hurt to be me. Why so much fear and pain? I had no answers, no justifications like all the grown-ups always seemed to have. The next best thing was to fight with all my might. The big yellow bus rolled into view in a flash and squeaked to a dusty stop.

Shit, I thought as my brothers and sisters walked towards the bus.

My mother said, "Come on now, put your rain coat on, Pauli, it is supposed to pour today."

"I really don't feel like going to school, Mom."

"Come on, Paul. Get on that bus."

This type of chatter went on for a few minutes while everyone in the school bus was gazing at me, wondering what my problem was.

My mother, fed up, screamed, "I have had enough, Paul! You are getting on that bus!"

I kicked and screamed as she dragged me and my ugly orange raincoat towards the bus. We reached the bus; she lifted me up and held me in while the bus driver tried to shut the door. It shut.

They were both much bigger than me and it did not take them very long to get their way. I was putting up a good old-fashioned hysterical fight.

They were obviously flustered. I was down in the stairwell with my fists pounding and pushing at the locked door that opened in the opposite direction of my force. I watched my mother cry, I cried, and the bus rolled towards school with a bunch of kids, my brothers and sisters, who all thought that I was totally nuts.

Scared and alone, I wondered what I had to do to make it better. I could not get away from the fact that my mother was bigger, the bus driver was much, much bigger and the teachers were bigger, too.

Sometimes my mother would give in and keep me home. That felt better than being at school but it did not feel good either. It was always a lie that got me there. I thought I was just a mother's boy and I guess she did, too. I slid through elementary school in this manner, not learning much of anything except that I was slow, a baby, a mother's boy, foul mouthed, a stupid, crazy kid on his way down. Myself, the teachers, my parents and some of my friends went right along with this half-spoken, half-sensed diagnosis.

# *Chapter 4*

## CAN YOU READ THE WRITING ON THE WALL

One of the nuns had read an article on dyslexia and she told my mother that I might "have it." It was about half way through the second grade when I started going to the "special school." I felt my parents' pain of having a child that did not fit in. It was obvious that things were more difficult for everyone involved. It's not easy jamming a square peg into a round hole.

"Why?" They would say, "we did everything, we gave you everything. Why don't you just do what you are supposed to do?"

"I'm not sure," I would say and think. I must be lazy.

The teachers' pain and frustration was evident also. I was still going to be attending the normal school full time. I only had to go to the special school for an hour after school; but to the teachers at the normal school, I was gone. I was somebody else's problem.

I never talked about the fact that I was having a hard time at school. To talk about it would be admitting that I was a problem. I did not want to be that much of a problem. I kept on looking for ways to hide or manipulate my way to get by. I blocked out everybody.

The summer had been carefree, but it never left the back of my mind that I still could not read. There was the "happy me" and the "scared me." What had happened in the second grade wound up happening again and again.

Once I got back to school I was spending more and more time eating soap and sitting in the principal's office. I was falling behind and being left behind in everything. The teachers would spend time with the kids who did not give them any trouble. I wanted to hide and the teachers did not want to see me. It seemed like they had been embarrassed by me too much and they just gave up. I was beginning to do the same. Trying to fit in was becoming too painful. If only I could have learned my multiplication tables.

At my desk looking out the window, I thought along with what I was learning in psychology and my research on learned helplessness. The helplessness was forming if not formed in those early years. This is going to take some serious work. Man, what the hell am I doing?

Back to the task. Another unsuccessful shot towards running. It's amazing how comfortable I am with the helplessness. Get to know your strengths, Paul, and focus on those.

NEEDING ANSWERS

Who will take the pain?
Is there anyone not in pain?
Who is left to take it?
Is it up to me?
No.
The pain goes on.
It flows and grows.
Generations in pain.

I know that it is up to me. But I'm not quite willing to accept that fact. I can not believe how comfortable I am in pain. Keep looking, Paul. Give it time.

Karafin was the name of the "special" school. I saw a lot of funny looking people there. I guess I must have been pretty funny looking myself. It was a school for the kids that did not fit into the normal school system. The school was only a short distance from my normal school. I walked there every day. I used to hate watching all the other kids go off on the buses, home to play, while I was on my way to try to read words being flashed on the wall faster and faster, so I could catch up.

They were projecting the words onto the wall and in time I was able to read them. What hurt was listening to the mumbles of the grown-ups behind closed doors. I was too afraid to ask them what was wrong with me. I could only imagine what they were saying about me. I could tell by the reactions at home and at school that the situation was not good at all.

"Why can't I just fit in? It would make it so much easier for everybody," I said to myself.

I got used to blocking things out in order to survive. It was easy to hide at home. There was always a lot going on. With four brothers and three sisters running around, doing their thing, I could get lost easily.

I wanted to be accepted, to be wanted, to be valued. The whole time I was questioning myself. I could see that I was different. I could feel that I was not getting what I needed but I thought it was my fault. I was on my own. The teachers at the normal school and my parents seemed to want to make believe that the problem was not there. That sounded like a good idea to me too.

One day as I walked to my special school, my dreams came true. Not the one about fitting in, but almost as good. I was sad, scared and down as usual when at school.  Walking with my head down, I passed the buses filled with happy kids laughing and screaming on their way home to play or just to get away.

Eddie, a friend of mine who walked home from school came running back to meet me screaming, "Paul, Paul your special school is blazing."

"Bullshit, leave me alone."

"No, no, I'm serious man, the school is torching."

"Come on Eddie, cut the crap."

"Follow me man, I'm serious, it's torching!"

I followed him as we ran around the corner.  I felt a huge sense of relief as I saw the dark, black smoke billowing from my special school.  Seeing the flames popping out of smashed windows felt even better.  My first thought was that I would be able to go home on the bus with the normal kids, at least for a while.

The fire fighters were trying to get some of the file cabinets out of the smoldering school.  I walked around the smoky, wet street checking out the scene. There were file cabinets strewn all over the sidewalk across the street.  I noticed a particular file cabinet, my special needs teacher's.  She had a big bag of bubble gum in the bottom drawer.  She would give me a piece or two if I was good.  I ducked under the commotion and opened the drawer. I was right, and it wasn't even all gooey from the heat.  I grabbed a handful, gave a bunch of pieces to Eddie, and walked away.

Because of all the traffic and commotion in town, my bus was still there.  I hopped on and went home to play and to get away.

I never mentioned the special school again. As far as I know nobody else did either. I did not want to go back. I wanted to fit in at any cost. I had learned a little from reading the words flashed on the wall, enough to slide by anyway, enough

18

to keep trying to fit in. It seemed like my parents wanted to go along with my manipulations too. They saw the pain I was going through. I was the only one out of the nine children who had a problem in school. They could not understand it. They did not want to believe it. My teachers could not understand it or control it either. Again the easiest thing to do was ignore it. We all silently agreed.

# *Chapter 5*

## THE DRASTIC CHANGE
## IT'S SAFE TO BE A STONE BUT IT'S HARD TO MOVE AROUND

The fourth grade was when I brought all my fear, anger and pain inward to another dimension. I brought it inward while I spat it outward as a diversion, an unconscious diversion which isolated me even more. I was feeling the world like a blow to the face on a freezing day.

I learned that being bad was a good distraction and attention grabber. I was becoming more and more frustrated and began to swear. Because of my swearing at the nuns and for some of my other distractions, I gained the respect from the bad boys. They did not fit in, and they could see that I did not, either.

Being bad led to dreaded talks with Dad. If I was "in deep" at school, he thought he had better give me a lecture. I was always telling the nuns to buzz off. It threw them. So I could hide the fact that I was different, maybe even dumb. And also in meeting my dad at least there was contact, even though one-sided. He would move into the library after dinner to do his homework. I would join him after he was in place.

"So," he would say. "Here you are again. Why is it that you insist on disobeying me? The rules are very clear. There is the right way and the wrong way. You consistently choose to go your own way, the wrong way."

"I'm just trying to find my way, Dad."

"Well, you had better start flying straight."

"Yeah, right." I would say under my breath, exiting silently.

I was one of the guys on their way down before they opened their mouths. Maybe it was the part of town that they were from. Maybe it was the clothes they wore, or the length of their hair, the color of their skin; who the hell knows? We had some sort of common ground to make communication possible. Maybe it was that some of our stresses were similar. Even though I felt pretty scared and uncomfortable, I started turning "being bad" into fun and found it was a great way to get around the reality of being left out. Maybe I could save some face. My self-esteem was getting shot at and hit every day. I had to have some way to cover. Being bad seemed to work.

My self-esteem was still getting knocked, but at least there was a reason for it, that I could somewhat understand. The attention that I was getting from the grownups in my life seemed to be a little less brutal, a little less threatening. Being bad was where it was at. That was easy enough. Maybe I would make it!?

Back at my desk trying to find some peace in the trees. I am angered at what our society is doing. It is plain and simple crap. We should know better. But what the hell can I do?

On second thought, I can see how it could just go on and on just by looking at how difficult it is for me to change myself. After walking down a destructive road for so long, what I can do to myself is just as much crap. Don't fight society, Paul. Just work on yourself now. I know. I need to get it all clearer in my mind. Be willing to be.

The negativity was growing on me like a vine twisting up on a great oak, slowly sapping its life. If the vine was given time to grow strong, it would choke the oak to a slow death, a death that would be difficult to see if one were not aware of what a vine can do when left to twist and curl with each passing day around a defenseless oak.

*"What is that around you?" said the little oak.*

*"It is me, it is part of me, little one. You see? You have one too. It is just the way it is."*

*"It looks like it is squeezing you! And mine is beginning to bother me, I think!"*

*"Ya, but it is just the way it is. I am used to it. It does not hurt anymore. I have accepted it."*

*"Are you sure it is part of you? It really doesn't look like it is."*

*"Just shut up, you are really beginning to bother me."*

I was seven and I was on my way. The next ten years were filled with the frustration of trying to fit into a system that did not work for me. The vine was growing fast. I had no idea what was happening to me. Each year the vine would grow and twist around me making sure it had a good strong hold. It was just the way it was. I was reinforcing the negative with almost every move I made. But by then the helplessness was well in place. Building on its own, sort of like a snowball rolling down a hill on a sticky, snowy day.

Looking back, falling into the helplessness took time. It was as if when I was young I was on top of a mountain looking west on a warm and windy summers day.

23

I could see thunderheads in the distance floating my way, flashing. I could also see shades of blue, purple, violet and red with the sun's thousands of reflections. The scenery is exciting and inviting.

As I climb down towards the valley the darkness builds. During the decent I lose sight of the diversity and brilliance. The gray reaches all the way down as the rain begins to fall.

All my report cards looked pretty much the same. They all were mediocre. Sometimes I was able to pull off a B. Most of the time it was a C. Sometimes it was the dreaded D. Even worse was the F. Failure, Jesus I had to stay away from that. But in some circles the crappy C was just as bad. And with the way I spelled there was no getting away from that.

In the effort section of the grades I would get torn apart, too. EFFORT includes: attempting to achieve learning goals, showing initiative in seeking assistance, having a positive attitude toward studies, completing assigned work, using time and materials wisely. P indicates a child's work is in proportion with his or her potential. M indicates the work is acceptable, but more effort is needed to achieve potential. L indicates work that it is even further below potential.

I never got a P; it was all Ms and Ls. I tried hard as hell to keep up, to not have to get the seemingly constant lectures on how being average will just not cut it in today's society of overachievers.

I truly thought that. I was lazy, I was stupid, I was bad.

What the hell was I going to do?

What was going to become of me?

24

With every period of the school year, the days absent were beginning to increase.

"If you do not start trying, you are going to wind up being a garbage man," said my mother out of the black.

A garbage man; what does that mean? Am I that bad? No, I don't think so, I thought to myself.

These people do not know what they are talking about. I am fine...? Well..., I am not sure.

Could they be right?

"Yeah right, Mom," I said as I walked away wishing I was somebody else.

What the hell is all this crap? I asked myself again while watching the trees outside. No one cares. How could they care? I do not even know how to get a point across on paper. The computer helps incredibly, but I need more help. There is no point to this.

Come on, Paul! Reality check; remember to look at the positive, the good. Look at what you have accomplished already. Sure there is still no black and white. It is hard to not have a clear and definite answer, but that is okay, that is life. You are slowly, through writing, getting honest with yourself and that is what matters. Something will come out of all this. Be good to yourself! You deserve it! Push on.

I know the child that is still me needs support. I also know there is a time to be firm with myself. This helplessness has been dragging me around for long enough!

It would come together piece by piece and then float away as if it had never been seen. The negative script and the helplessness on top of it have a cunning way to make the problem worse as time goes by unless confronted. It is also something that I have been living with for a long time. It is going to take persistence and patience to change. I pushed on.

Remember that you need to confront the past. Just be. Affirm yourself for being you! Pull on.

This is much more than I thought it would be. I am bouncing around like a super ball.

Though I will not run out on myself again.


## CLOUDS

They come and go.
To where, from where,
No one really knows.
The sun is bright and warms to the bone.
In the shade there is a chill.
The wind blows, the leaves rustle,
Some float to the ground.
Others fall like stones.
The sun streams back in.


It is much safer, it is much easier, to fit in, to go along with the pack, not to make waves. I felt this at age two and sometimes still do. I believe all children feel it and thus strive to do and be the same as they see. All this makes for good survival tactics. If someone else did something one way and they lived, then their way works and that is the way it should be done. This all makes some sense; but it looks to me like we became lost in the safeness of it all. We became so lost that we cannot even see that "the way" does not work properly.  Our jails are full.  There is drug and alcohol abuse almost everywhere you look.  The school systems are in shambles.  Children are getting pregnant.  People are killing each other in record numbers.

I could go off on this mode forever; but the reality is that there is a need for me to get back to myself.  Taking the focus off me and looking at the whole world is just another way of setting myself up for failure.  The mode that I need to be in, is to risk growing, to really live free.  Changing one's life script is possible!  I can feel it.  Back to the past, to get a better grasp on the present.

# Chapter 6

## THE DESTRUCTIVE CIRCLE

I was in ninth grade. I did not go straight from St. Francis to Fordham Prep or JFK. I went back to another grammar school that "just happened" to have one extra grade. I stayed back, something I had always feared. It was like catching a bullet right between the eyes. I went down.

I still hated school with a passion. My Latin was poor, to say the least, which was made painfully obvious with more humiliation every day. I still could not read English well, let alone another language. I struggled to get by. Sooner, rather than later, final exam time would roll around and trash any positive record that I might have managed to build up.

As far as my teachers and parents saw it, I was not doing well enough to survive. My life script had been set. I was not asking myself, how far can these people see anyway? I was just giving in to the pain of not fitting in trying to figure out why; getting strokes and stroking myself whenever possible. The problem was that most of them were negative, reinforcing my bogus beliefs about who I was and what I could do.

What's the use? It just does not matter, nothing matters, this world is a bad joke.

During all this time I did have an outlet. I was able to experience successes in sports but even at this early stage of my life the negative force was powerful. It was much stronger and ingrained than the positive. I naturally excelled in sports; but without the belief that I was okay, worthy of success, I was doomed to mediocrity. The negative seemed now to be the only way I knew how to get the attention I needed. The invisible vine of negativity and helplessness was holding strong and growing fast. With every report card the drill followed about how lazy and unfocused I was. The good stuff never seemed to be good enough. I knew in a way that I was not stupid, but I could not hold on to this knowledge.

Sitting in study hall, late one fall looking at the Cs and Ds on my report card and knowing how my parents and teachers were going to react, I began to scribble and swear on the report card.

"You are so damn stupid! You are a lazy jerk. Why the hell are you so god damn dumb. Mom was right! The only thing you will be able to do with grades like these is be a garbage man."

I crumbled up the report and jammed it into my pocket and dreamed of walking alone through the fields back home listening to the wind howl and the birds sing or squawk.

That night the dinner table was crowded. My younger brother took out his report card and started showing it off. I am not knocking my brother. If I ever had a report that they would have been proud of I would have shown it off also.

My mother said, "Paul, where is your report card?"

I reached into my pocket forgetting about the swears I had written on it earlier. As I uncrumpled the report I saw the words.

I crumpled the report once again and replied, "I don't want to show it to you."

"You have to. Let me see it."

"No. It is just more of the same anyway."

As she reached across the table for it and me, I took off. I passed the garbage can and threw a crumpled up napkin in, to get her off my tail. It worked. She looked in the can, I proceeded on to the library bathroom and flushed the report card down the toilet. When I returned to the kitchen she had the napkin in her hand.

"See, you can be smart when you want to."

I went out for a walk through the field. I was down on myself. I could not hear the wind or the birds. The negative voice within was getting louder and louder blocking out the good like when the wind changes direction and sends the air traffic noise over your spot on the beach. The sound of the wind and waves get lost from time to time; but luckily they are always there.

I sat back from the keyboard. I needed to rest, take a look at the trees; and maybe after a while take a closer look at me. Looking back at this stuff really hurts sometimes. Doomed to mediocrity and not sure why; it's enough to make me cry. But now I am beginning to see; that is why the pain is so real. But it's okay. I do not have to let it stop me. There is air, clean air at the end of the tunnel. No need to hang and gag.

### UNREST

I would walk among the trees.
They would befriend me.
Humans I do not particularly like.

31

The days past.
Streams of light through the woods,
Help me to see,
what was passing in front of me.

There is a common insecurity in people. I thought, the ones who can accept this are the ones that do not go crazy trying to figure everything out. They have realistic goals for themselves and others. In some areas of life, there are no answers; there is no right or wrong. Becoming an individual, stepping out, is challenging. It is really living. To doubt, wonder and wish is real. It is human. Some day I will find my way. Back then it did not seem to matter much. Now it can and it does.

Go back.

The repetition might seem crazy to a reader; but you have to try and understand that I'm not trying to jam anything into anyone's head. I'm trying to push out the negative within myself. The spiral down has been long and it's ingrained.

Moving from the helplessness is like trying to climb back up that mountain. It is tough to get started on a dark and dismal day. But I remember a bit of what it is like at the top. With each step up my view widens. Though it is wet for a while I can sense that I will break through the clouds. Soon the sun will dry me. Soon I will see the colors again.

# Chapter 7

## TRAPPED

I made it from the Harvey School to Fordham Prep where two brothers before me had gone. I was going to have to be a freshman. Back another grade and that pissed me off; but I figured that it was worth it in order to look good to my family. Possibly it would keep me from a life of garbage.

I had made it to high school. I had not accomplished a damn thing. My self-esteem was still plummeting. I could feel it. The vine was still growing. I thought that was just the way it was for people who have a hard time getting through the school system. Fordham was a competitive high school, and I had no idea of what I was setting myself up for. I was even more determined to do it on my own. I was fifteen; I did not trust anybody, not even myself. To ask for help would be like calling myself stupid. Admitting that I do not have what it takes to fit in would be like saying, "okay, you parents and teachers are right. I am destined to be a garbage man." Although today being a garbage person is the thing to be. This world is so full of it you could become very successful in the eyes of the competition. But the message they were trying to convey, and did, was simply negative. Plus I was not trying to fit in for financial reasons. I was trying to fit in to find love.

It was during the year at Fordham that I found out what pot and cocaine could do for one's pain. When high, the pain would be gone. It would come back, however most of the time it would be a little worse. But I was high and forgetting my problems was my goal, not working on them. I had been working on my problems for a long time, ever since I entered school, most of my life. I was not only getting nowhere, but the problem was getting worse. When high, I felt no pain. My self-esteem was at a new low and the teachers and parents were not to be blamed. It was me now, on my own rolling down a destructive road of negativity feeding the vine that was killing me, throwing my self-esteem out the window and not knowing it.

English class at Fordham was intense. The teacher was also my homeroom mentor; he looked like Abe Lincoln, dark and stern with a warm side. The class and he scared the hell out of me.

I could understand well what was going on in class and I enjoyed part of it. Analyzing poems, songs and short stories that were read in class by people that were good at reading aloud was intriguing. But we also had to read outside of class and report back with a short written passage at the beginning of each class. The reading may have taken me longer than most but I usually had no problem getting cool points from them. When it came to getting the points I saw out on paper, what I wrote was unacceptable. The style was pretty much the same as this story, stabby and jumpy, tough to connect at times but most of the time the point did get across.

One of the big differences was the spelling. I couldn't and still can't spell. Now the computer spells for me. With hours of spell checking I can usually clean up a paper. I can see why my papers would be thrown away now but I did not understand then. It was clear that my work was bad. It was not clear why it couldn't be talked about. But after all how could one expect to get into an ivy league school with writing like that.

College was not the main thing on my mind. It was more important to make it through the day without getting laughed at. So I stopped doing the homework which lead to not not going to class which lead to blowing off school all together.

After failing at Fordham I went to a public high school. It was easy compared to Fordham. I did not feel like I was being attacked every day. There was mediocrity that I could get lost in. There were people worse off than I. Part of me took on the mind set of the parent-teacher and just gave up on myself. Another part of me kept on fighting; but now that I had drugs on my side, my chances were getting slimmer and slimmer every day. The situation was already as fragile as driving down a bumpy road with a jar of nitro. I decided to go four-wheeling.

It was a crisp, cold spring evening. There was an immense amount of life at the party on the old Indian reservation, deep in the back woods of Westchester. Everyone was festive and lively.

I was deep in thought. Gazing into the large camp fire, I could not help thinking about how the native Americans must have felt two hundred years ago, pushed onto, trapped in a new life that they hated with a passion. The Natives had been trapped and pushed around by the white man, who did not even know their language, much less their culture. The white man thought he was better. He thought he was God, and that his system was the only system. The white man feared what he could not or would not try to understand.

It is a cold and lonely feeling to be so totally controlled by people who seem only to care for the system; how they look in it and to it. The more I related to the lost culture of the native Americans, the more I could feel my body beginning to tense up.

It was after nine. I was feeling disconnected and not sure why. Maybe it was because I knew I was supposed to have had the Jeep home by nine. Maybe I felt different all the time because of the anger that had built up inside while trying to conform. Maybe I was just bad. I lost touch with reality, if I ever knew what reality was. I could not see a way to escape the twisted feeling. The mortal gods, parents, teachers and self were in control. I was too scared to not have an answer.

That night there were no drugs; so excitement was what I was after. I went for a joy ride with four young women from the party. We went four-wheeling with my Jeep in the black woods of the reservation. Returning to the main road, I was seen by a cop at the other end of a long straightaway. The flashing, blue lights seemed to be in a fog as they were gaining on me in slow motion.

My calf muscle tensed as I hit the gas. Was it my drive for excitement, or could I just not deal with grown-ups anymore? Why was everything always in the fog? The Jeep roared away. My leg now locked in a position with the accelerator to the floor. The girls screamed to stop me, but I blocked out even my best friends' pleas.

I had outrun the cops before and thought I could get away with it again. There was a ninety-degree turn at the exit of the reservation. The Jeep could not hold the curve. The back end slid out and crushed a guard post. Compressed air began to hiss from a leak in the right rear tire. I cruised at speeds of sixty to eighty MPH down the winding, country road leading away and to the next town.

The cops, now in force, were screaming and screeching in hot pursuit. Before each turn I looked back, to see if I could get around a turn without being seen. I made one but kept on speeding down the road anyway. The next turn was a sharp left, I turned to the left side of the road in order to give the Jeep more road to skid around the turn. Before we even got to the turn the Jeep was on its side. The speed and the now flat right rear tire flipped it. Sparks were flying everywhere as if we were in a war zone. The sound of metal scraping along the pavement was a horrid sound that seemed to go right through me. The Jeep went straight off the road on its side, and up a steep hill at seventy plus. We hit a boulder and flipped nose to tail. I smashed through the windshield, feet first. Before I had been totally thrown from the vehicle, the Jeep landed on its roof and pinned me. It rolled back down the hill and stopped silently in the middle of the road. No one made a sound.

I was trapped, crushed between the dashboard and the roof. At first I did not realize how stuck I was, nor was there any pain. I shook the girls. All of them were curled up in a ball, by my side, still none of them making a sound. After I shook them they began to scream again.

I yelled, "get out, get out!" They crawled out of the twisted wreck to safety, screaming and crying in fear and confusion. When I tried to move, I realized how pinned I was. I lost control. I didn't want to die. When the first cop arrived he yelled at me, breaking me away from my fear.

"You have to turn the car off." The cop yelled.

"I can't reach the key."

"You have to reach it. Try."

"Just get the car off me." I screamed.

"I'm not Herculean, kid. Turn it off!"

In reaching to turn it off I had to stretch and in doing so I dislocated my shattered hips. The pain knocked me out, but the Jeep was off. When I passed out, the girls thought I had died. There were no sounds at all coming from the crushed Jeep. It was peaceful. I could feel no pain. I felt more peaceful then I could ever remember feeling. In my dream there was no one to bother me, not even myself.

When I awoke there was a fireman crouched beside me with a saw and a knife. The knife he used to cut off my faded jacket.

"Jesus, I thought you were dead," said the fireman.

"No, not yet," I said and smiled weakly.

The fireman proceeded to use the saw to cut some metal away, so he could fit the Jaws of Life in place. It was past eleven before the fireman could start the painful, tedious procedure. They had to change the pressure on my body slowly or my insides would have burst like a balloon with too much air in it.

By this time there was a large crowd of people on the normally deserted road. The tension was high as a tow truck pulled near, backfiring loudly. The paramedics and firemen scattered. Just at that moment the Jaws of Life began to free me. My breathing was slowly getting easier as centimeter by centimeter the pressure on me lessened. My god, I was going to make it out of this mess. I enjoyed the free breathing and tried to drag myself out. A young woman from the crowd saw me struggling, and she ran over and dragged me out. The paramedics were a little pissed but they were too busy strapping me to a board to acknowledge it.

I was trapped again and screaming in agony.

"No please, I said leave my legs bent."

"We can't."

"Jesus Christ, you have got to let me leave them bent."

"It's procedure. We have to strap you down so you can't move."

"No way." I said as I swung with whatever strength I had and caught the paramedic with a right hook to the jaw. The next thing I knew they had me strapped at the ankles, knees, waist, wrists, chest and forehead. They had me. I screamed. My body had become used to the distorted configuration in which the twisted metal had me. My body went cold. I asked them to warm me, but no amount of blankets could. I shivered and cried for I did not want to die. Trapped.

Later in the hospital I realized that I was lucky to be alive, though part of me really did not care that much. I was grateful that none of the girls or any innocent bystanders were hurt. If they had, I don't think I would be here today.

For most of the month -- my long stay at the hospital -- I was high on demerol, a powerful pain killer. I felt no pain at all, physical or mental. The communication with parents was pretty much non-existent and, like so many times in the past, it seemed that not talking about a problem would make it go away. Time was sliding by. I left the hospital with a pocket full of the wrong prescriptions; and went back home with even more emotional pain.

I had a tutor at home to help me catch up so I could finish my sophomore year at high school. I was pretty much high the whole time as I lay in bed with this bald headed freak sitting by, telling me that I was just a C student. That was all there was to it.

One afternoon my oldest brother entered the room to bring us some tea.

After the bald-headed freak had spoken with him for a few minutes he pronounced knowingly, "you are a B+ student."

My brother said, "What?"

"You are a B+ student, am I right?"

My brother proudly said, with a smile on his face, "yes, that's right."

The freak turned back to me and said, "You see, I have had a lot of experience with students. I can see what they are capable of just by speaking with them."

I thought to myself. The freak was right about my brother. HE must be right about me. More of the same, what the hell is going to become of me? This school thing is still getting worse. Aaaa, it doesn't matter anyway.

The beat went on. I needed someone to help me. I did not trust anyone enough to ask. My environment was negative, my only friends were the pain killers. They soon started to cause much more pain than they killed.

# *Chapter 8*

## COMMUNICATE DON'T MEDICATE

I am sitting at the computer and my body feels like jumping out of its skin. When in pain, I look to the trees. Their calming colors, along with the gentle breezes help to bring me back to the here and now only to leave once again in a story of roots, vines and branches. But I seem to be more willing or better able to start placing myself in the forest, clinging to the more familiar.

*The forest was infested with strong vines and no one knew it. Everybody was being stunted. Stunted was all they seemed to know. All the young were looking up to the towering elders, vines and all, some trying desperately to fit in and be just like them. It seemed safe, the approval felt life giving.*

*The trees were not talking much, everyone was trying to go along. Some could not do it. They tried to rely on their roots but their leaves kept on telling them to conform. They sprouted with the soil, sun and rain but now believed they needed the system to survive and be loved.*

Trying to get back to the task. I know these vines of learned helplessness are still around me. Change is frightening; it is like climbing high in a tree and suddenly the wind begins to rise. The tree sways and so do I. I have a firm grip on the limb but it is not the same as the larger limb below with the vines that I can slide my hand underneath to further support me in case the wind continues to rise.

Again I think about climbing back down onto the strangely comforting limb of negativity and thus failure. The child in me is scared; scared of the unknown upper limbs. To trust the upper limbs it is going to take a patient and persistent parent within to reassure the frightened child. It is important that we are not hurried. It is important to see that it is important. While the other parent within is telling me that I am useless.

### FEAR

> Blue and green,
> Are the colors,
> Today.
> Sad, but growing.
> Scared,
> Not knowing.

As I grew it became more and more obvious, even with my manipulations, that I was not performing at an acceptable level. My need to fit in at any cost was changing. A price in pain was obvious. I tried to talk, and I tried again and again, but my nature was to fight.

I had again to save face and the easiest words to use, the ones that came out most often when I was extremely frustrated, scared, and in pain, were obscenities. The sad thing was that becoming the kid that swore and acted out all the time was once again a defeatist move. It made it easy for me to walk away. Saying to myself, it just does not matter, they will never understand me.

On the other hand it also made it easy for the adult to write me off as having a behavioral problem. It got them off the hook and in turn added a whole new dimension in the knocking of my self-esteem. I was reinforcing the life script of being a bad person with no real chance of ever fitting in, being accepted, being loved.

### CHANGE

The air is heavy but cool.
The fall is near.
Looking forward to the change.
The evergreen doesn't seem to notice.

*The oak said to the evergreen, "How can you bear the weight of the snow when it falls? I am glad I lose my leaves come fall. For if I didn't my branches would snap."*

*"I am made up of soft flexible wood. You are made up of hard wood. We are different."*

*"Oh yeah, that is right. We are different."*

Back to the task. I feel better. I am not alone. I see people getting nailed and nailing themselves all over the place. Scared to speak out, afraid to be. If I show the real me and I get put down again, what the hell will happen to me? Who the hell knows? I do know that it is better to go for it. I have to.

After a while, the pills slowed my mind and body to the point of total and utter despair. I was complaining of headaches that would just not go away. My

43

mother set up an appointment at a hospital so my brain could be scanned. I was slow from the drugs and didn't figure that she would trick me. I walked with her into the mental hospital still not knowing what it was. Three men in white coats told my mother to leave. I could see her crying through the small window of the heavy steel door as she walked backwards, away. The men in the white coats told me to empty my pockets and take all my clothes off. I fought for a week straight. I was trapped again. I would not accept it at all. I was either fighting with all my might, crying in the pain of being alone, or too exhausted or drugged to move at all.

After several days of fighting they shot me up with a heavy dose of pheno-barbital. As the hours passed I felt my strength coming back. I rolled off the bed onto the floor and started doing push ups in hopes of wearing the drug off faster. It worked. I was ready to fight again, though I lay in bed acting as if I could not move.

The doctor entered saying, "Paul, why do you insist on fighting us? We are trying to help you."

"Ya right," I said, as I sat up.

The doctor, with a surprised look on his face, started backing towards the door. He was halfway out as I darted towards the door that he was trying to close behind him. I leaped at the door karate style and kicked the heavy wooden door shut. When I opened the door, I saw the doctor sprawled on the floor. I ran to the far end of the hall and tried to rip the wire fence from the window. It was hopeless; there was no way. When I turned there were three more attendants with white coats coming down the hall towards me. I ran straight at them full speed. As we clashed I caught one of them in the jaw with all the weight and speed behind my tightly clenched fist. I broke through them without losing much speed at all, but there was still the steel door at the end of the hall to contend with.

I was desperate. I did not have the keys. I had no rights at all. I tried to take my weight and speed through the door. I hit the floor in pain, as my legs and hips, still fragile from the accident, buckled as I hit the door. Even if I had been operating at full strength, my legs still would have buckled. The guys in the white coats carried me back to my room. The largest of the three held me by the collar once I was lying in bed.

He said, "Paul, stop fighting, man. Stop fighting. If you keep this crap up, you may never get out of here."

There was something about that guy's face or maybe it was the caring tone in his voice. Anyway, somehow he reminded me of a friend. I stopped fighting.

I was scared out of my mind. I was still trapped. At seventeen I had no rights at all, the only change was that I stopped fighting. I spent another week and a half at the mental hospital. They gave me all sorts of tests. One of their main findings was the fact that I was dyslexic. One of the doctors told me that the dyslexia could explain my frustration, anger and acting out.

She said, "Most kids who go undetected all the way to 17 are either in jail, a drug addict, dead or of course any combination of the three."

I thought to myself, Great! An answer!

I knew that drugs were not going to be able to help me learn more about dyslexia or help me get out of the jam I was in. Drugs were only good for running or dying. I had a spark to go on.

One of the other great revelations at the hospital was that I needed a place to go. I didn't need to be locked up listening to screams in the night and watching people walk around like zombies because for them to quietly fit in, they needed (or the system needed) to give them daily voltage.

With all the games, manipulations, misunderstandings, and confusion, home was looking just as bad as the hospital, if not worse.

Where can I go? I thought along with the doctor.

The next night I was awakened by what sounded like a dying person's screams, they echoed through the halls for hours. I didn't know what to do. And I couldn't fall back to sleep. A few days later I saw a gorgeous girl. She was beautiful. I had to talk with her.

"Hi," I said tentatively.

"Hi," she replied.

It was a beautiful day outside and both of us could not help to recognize it. After talking with her for awhile I found out that the room she had come from was padded and that this was the first time that she had been out since both her parents were killed in a plane accident. She had been the one screaming in the night.

"It is so nice out. Can we go outside?" she said.

"I can't, but you probably could. Ask that guy over there."

"Can I go out for a walk?" she asked.

"Are you kidding? No way. You have been a bad girl," the guard said. She pleaded, but to no avail.

"Why can't you let her take a short walk?" I asked.

"It's none of your god damn business," the guard said.

I said, "You're an idiot, man."

"What?"

"You heard me. You're a fool."

He leaped up to contain me but it was too late. I was off and running again, looking for any way to escape. The next thing I knew I was fighting again. It was the same losing battle. I wound up confined to my room. It didn't matter, though. I was better off not having to watch what was going on. I never saw the girl again, but I think of her often.

In time I calmed down, though it wasn't easy to get out. I thought that I had support from the doctor. But he just faded into the woodwork like every other adult I knew. The doctor knew as well as I that if he was going to help it was going to take standing up to the parents. He changed his mind without informing me. For him to help he would have had to confront the almighty parents and the almighty school system.

In my mind I was saying, Paul, forget it man, just get the hell out of this place before they decide that the easiest thing to do would be to shock my brain until I am what they want me to be.

When my mother came to bring me home, she was all smiles and tense hugs like nothing ever happened. It did not matter because everything was going to be fine.

I felt free. I could feel the breeze in my face, and the strong sun as we drove home in silence.

This part brought up some pain and anger. I was looking at the trees and listening to the neighbor's dog yap. I wanted to kill that dog.

But it is not the dog, it's the master. How the hell can people leave a dog chained all day on a ten-foot line? It makes me want to go chain up the owners and see how they like it.

Though now I look back at a poem I wrote earlier.

### UNREST

I would walk among the trees.
They would befriend me.
Humans I do not particularly like.
The days past.
Streams of light through the woods.
Help me to see.
What was passing in front of me.

I am human too and though I don't understand what we are capable of doing at times it can't help to hate myself. I will get nowhere with that. Sometimes I wonder if I have enough patience and persistence in me.

### TO BE

Different
First fear
Then proud
To stand among others
To become
ME

I always had my roots, but I did not listen to them much. When I did they would just say that I was okay and they helped me make it to another day.

**LIFE**

Living in the day.
Once the jump has been made,
It's up to the wind.
There is no way back.
In freedom there is fear.

# *Chapter 9*

## CLIMBING WITHOUT A HOPE

As soon as I arrived home from the hospital, I packed my bags and walked across town to my girlfriend's house. She seemed to love me and her parents did, too. I spent about six months with them. John Lennon was shot and killed. I worked in a small camping gear shop. I tried to sort out some of my pain and confusion and soon realized that things still looked pretty bleak. I loved my girlfriend and her family. They were caring and nice. I was sad to leave them but I was still being driven by the need to conform, read, write, get good grades, find love at home. Then and only then would I feel at ease.

If I go back to school, I thought, then I will be accepted. Somehow.

It was another special school. It was a co-ed boarding school, this time, in northwestern Connecticut, The Forman School, a beautiful spot to be, though my stomach never felt that good when in the vicinity of a school. And this school I would be living at.

It did not take me very long to fit in with the wild crowd. The kids who loved to live on the edge, giving the teachers something to do with their rules of power and control if they could catch us. I met many misfits like myself at this school. We did manage to have some good times. But there were still negative messages. There was not enough communication or just plain miscommunication about what the problems actually were. For a place highly regarded as being one of the best in helping people with learning differences, the school was a big disappointment. Anyone could see, even if blind, that the varying degrees of school-related and or behavioral problems needed to be talked about; but this school was trying to look like a major league prep school. It had the land. It had the buildings with ivy growing up the walls. It even had the teachers with their bow ties, corduroy blazers and accents from some unknown planet of their own far, far away from the needs of the students. What the needs were I had no idea at the time. But I knew something was wrong.

My first report card brought it all back to me. Average effort B-student. I could easily account for the B's because I was at a "special" school. My father helped me to see this.

"You see, son. Things would be a lot harder at Fordham, or in the real world. You had better get in gear or you will be left behind. How are you going to survive then?"

I would say to myself as I walked away or hung up the telephone, I don't know, I just do not know???

God damn it, this school is supposed to be for people like me. I still can't fit in.

If I did, it would not really matter anyway.

This is not the real world.

Where is the real world?

Is there one?

I hope I can find it some day!

Back to my writing room, my plants, my pictures, my music, and the trees outside my window. Learning how to give myself a break, that is all. Simple but hard.

"The Real World," and what a world it is. If one attempts to take it all in, to really look at how much sense the real world makes, one becomes so depressed one does not even bother trying to change. Some see the deterioration and ugliness as normal or to just be the way that it is.

Well if this is the way it is, then I can't continue to believe what they say when they and me, tell me that I'm bad, that I'm wrong, that there is no better way, because our perspective is twisted.

I don't think they know; and if I keep trying to live up to these expectations I could die. And I don't deserve to die. I have something very important to say.

Today, I must go on.

My world I can do something about. I know now I can do something. I'm doing it.

All right, Paul, back to Forman. What happened?

My self-esteem was lower, but in order to try and hide that fact and prevent it from continuing to dive into a black hole, I went right back to the "all-out bad boy" routine. Skipping class, cutting on teachers whenever possible, not bothering with trying, and doing bong hits whenever possible were my usual activities. It just did not matter.

I met a girl at this school. It was a special time in my life. She was just as wild as I. We had a blast getting into trouble together. Everyone knew that I was always up to something but they never actually did catch me. My speed came in handy. I made it through the school year without getting kicked out. It was another year of reinforcing my negative life script. It was no great achievement except for the fact that I did manage to stay alive, not living but surviving.

One of my friends killed himself, a bullet in the head. I could not understand a pain that bad or I just could not handle thinking about it. I just walked on. I was watching life pass like day into night on a dark cloudy day.

That summer I was out west with some friends riding in the mountains of Montana when I received a frantic call from my mother.

"Paul, your headmaster called. He said that you have been kicked out of school. He wouldn't give me an explanation as to why. I could not believe it. You are my son. I have a right to know. Do you know what is going on?"

"I have no idea, Mom." But I knew, and my whole body began to shake. My voice cracked as I tried to end the conversation.

"You have to come home right now and straighten this all out."

"All right," I said and hung up the phone.

I knew that my girlfriend was pregnant and that an abortion had been planned. Somebody just found out or something else went wrong. I was too scared to find out. I was frozen with the fear of the unknown until I arrived home a day later.

My girlfriend was as fine, as fine could be considering the intensity of the situation; and to top it off having to deal with the school and parents as well as with life and death. Somehow the school nurse had found out and reported it. My girlfriend's mother was great and helped her get through all the pain and confusion. The school did not say anything about kicking her out, but they wanted me out.

I drove up to have a "little chat" with the headmaster to find out what he thought my options were and to get a quick look at what they were.

"Welllllllll Paul," he said, "as I see it you have three options."

"#1 You can tell your parents and leave the school."

"#2 You can not tell your parents and leave the school."

"#3 You can come back to the school but you will not be able to be seen with your girlfriend at all."

I thought to myself. This is a small school, I love my girlfriend, and I am not fast enough to pull it off. The whole thing will be even more of a bad game than it already is. What about #4, none of the above? I thought.

"You have got to be kidding."

"No, I am not Mr."

"Fine, later, much later. I guess it really will be none of the above." I drove home wondering what the hell I was going to do next.

When I told my mother what was going on she could not believe it. She is a very strict Catholic. In her eyes I had made the worst possible move that I ever could have and, indeed, in my own eyes.

"Do not tell anybody about this, not a soul," she advised.

I said to myself, Wowww, this is great. I do not have to talk about this ever again. This is much easier then I thought it was going to be.

"Ok, Mom," I replied and left the cool, dark room with a sigh, a mixed bag of a sigh.

## UNCERTAINTY

Uncertainty
Silence in a storm,
Like peace in confusion.
Peaceful for a time,
The gusts move in,
Vision is fogged.


The flames were low but the coals were glowing as the hard wood crackled and smoked. I was feeling blue and the feeling was growing, because of my overblown need to try to control the uncontrollable. I let it grow, like a forest fire burning out of control, on a blistering, dry summer's day. Could I slow the blaze down, or put a stop to it? Is it the forest's time to crackle and crumble? Time to burn out the thick dark woods, where the strong, well-planted vines are slowly choking the life out of many of the trees. The struggling trees stand there half dead, blocking the sun from the new trees trying desperately to emerge. Should I stop trying to fight the blaze, and let it burn, burn out of control? How much control do I have anyway?

While the forest dies slowly, it prevents so many potential trees from a chance to feel the sun. It is part of nature's cycle for forests to burn sometimes. The white pine tree's seeds do not have a chance to germinate unless the cones are burned, forcing them to open, springing new life through death. A brand-new chance for growth in a dead-looking, burned-out forest, once ruled by the vines.

I will take a risk and let the fire burn. I have to have faith that a new forest will come.

But when will it come?

How long will it take to grow?

So many fears, not enough answers.  Faith, faith is much better than a slow, painful death trying to control a wild fire.


**ACCEPTANCE**

Anything will grow now.
Now that change is possible.
Renewal,
Every day,
Every  year,
Every second.
One story leads to another.
Sight or insight?
It is seeing just the same.

## *Chapter 10*

## I'M GONE

It was on to another school. Where was it going to be? What sort of image would come along with it? Would the school help? Could it help?

My parents said that they found a great school for me in Florida; that it was time for me to pack my bags. I was happy to be packing. With all the bad things I had done, I figured they really did not want me around anyway.

The school was in the middle of Florida. It was not on the ocean like I had been hoping, but there was a big lake.

All right I thought, they have a ski boat. This could be hot.

Then I found out that it was hot; not the same hot that I was thinking about, but hot as hell. It was so hot that you couldn't swim in the lake. Because when the water got too warm, a fungus would grow. If you were swimming, this fungus could enter through your nose and eat your brains.

"I came all this way. Let's look at the rest of the school," I said doubtfully.

We walked around the school. My fear was growing with each room that we entered. Kids were saying stuff that did not make any sense. One of them was screaming. There had to "be a reason." We went on to look at the dorms. They were not pretty; they didn't look comfortable at all. It didn't look like a helpful place.

I told my parents and the dude showing us around, "there is not a chance in hell that I am going to stay. If you do not want to take me home, that's fine, I will hitch hike, I will do what ever it is that I have to do. I am not staying here."

The teachers and my parents went behind closed doors to discuss my fate as I sat outside in the blistering heat wondering if they could force me to stay.

I turned eighteen this year, they can't make me do a god damn thing. I breathed a sigh of relief and waited to see what they had to say. I was not sure if I could make it out of this orange-infested area. And I would only strike out on my own if I had to. It would be a hell of a lot easier if they flew me somewhere, anywhere but here. It was too damn hot.

They came out from behind the door and my father said, "I guess this is not such a great place for you after all. Let's go home." He bought another ticket for me. We were soon in the air.

It was late in the day and the sun was beginning to set when we took off into the sky. There was a thunder storm with amazing bolts of lightning to the south west. The sun setting in the west caught some of the rain and darkness from the storm. It made one of the most incredible scenes I had ever witnessed, a rainbow in the sunset with a storm either coming or going. I was glad to be in the air.

It is disgusting how dependent I was. I look back at this stuff and sometimes it really blows my mind. Even now I wonder why I put myself through so much hell.

Then I have to remember that it took years of negative affirmations from parents, teachers, and self. I had no clue who or where I was. In reality, how could I expect it of myself at that age with all those strikes against me to just step out on my own and follow the positive force from within?

Just get it out, Paul. The past is gone. It is a done deal. What you have to do is deal with now, today. That is all you have.

*Everyone was gone. It all started when the visitors arrived unannounced. It was slow at first but once a few had been taken it spread like wild fire.*

*It was very hard to tell the difference between one that was real and one that was gone. And soon being gone was the norm. It was the easiest way to live.*

*Fighting the gone didn't work. The only way you could help one that was gone was to not be gone yourself. Remember to stick close to those you know are not gone. If you are on your own you can be easily sucked into the gone's way of life. The gone are powerfully subtle manipulators. The gone will do anything to hold on to their way; for if they lose that, they feel they will lose everything. Tips for approaching the gone. Shock them with kindness. They need to see us treat each other well. They need to see a reason to come back.*

# *Chapter 11*

## SOMEONE TO RELY ON

I needed to graduate from a high school and the doctor at the Karafin school came to my rescue. One year at Karafin and I would get the piece of paper that I desperately needed, a high school diploma. Dr. Greenfelt knew what the problem was. He accepted me for what I was. We worked from there. He was a friend of mine. Just being around someone who showed some acceptance without condescension took a load of worries off my mind.

I was able for the first time in my life to take a test untimed so I might better show what it was that I knew. The classes were small which made it difficult for me to get lost. I was getting tired of fighting. I was trying to get lost less.

I was getting help and doing well. I achieved As and Bs at Karafin; but again it really did not matter. I was taking these tests untimed. In the real world nothing is done untimed.

The fight was to go on. How else was I ever going to be accepted? My college plans were grand. I would do a double major in Finance/Banking and Social Psych with the final objective of a doctorate. One of my career interests was real estate. Somehow I was going to put the past behind me, go off on my own, be fine and make it big.

It was on to a small reputable college in Vermont where one of my sisters had gone. By this time it was well known to me that I would be needing some help, but I really did not want to admit it. It still meant degradation. But, officials at the school said they were familiar with the problem and that they could help. It was the easiest next step for me to make in order to keep trying to fit in. I had graduated in December from high school, but I didn't attend the ceremony. My father went and accepted the diploma for me.

So I had some free time before September. I set out with a couple of hundred bills to a small island off the east coast where there were hard labor jobs. I landed a job with a builder and went right to work. It felt good waking with the sun every day and working until it went down. It felt good learning new things every day, working physically and not being put down. I managed to save enough money to move out of the boarding house, and rented a house with a friend. It was a big house and eventually I had to call some old friends and have them come help us pay the summer rent and have a good time.

My boss was a tough Irish man who was very successful but obviously working himself into an early grave. He was a respected man who had already had one heart attack and acted like he was looking forward to the next. He could not enjoy the riches he had worked for. There was always more to be done, more respect to be gained.

He had a small biplane that he would take out before the sun had a chance to rise for a little excitement. He dared me to meet him at the airport one morning. I accepted with a nervous smile. He warned me not to eat breakfast.

You couldn't see the sun but you could tell it was going to show itself within the next fifteen or twenty minutes. We each grabbed a wing and rolled the plane out of its hangar. He started it, warmed it up, and we took off five minutes to spare before the sun shone painfully over the surface of the water. I forgot to bring shades.

He tried to scare the hell out of me and he did. I tried to hide the fear. I was well practiced at that and did a fairly good job. The G force gauge in front of me was shooting back and forth as he laughed hysterically. The sun coming up seemingly out of the ocean was now blinding. It was hard to breathe hanging from the seat harness. When we came around to an upright, level flying position, I had time to catch my breath. Then I thought of this guy's heart and imagined splashing into the fiery water. I thought I could hear my heart over the loud hum of the engine right in front of my face with my red-faced boss at the stick behind me laughing.

"You have to land this baby at a high speed or you risk nosing into the runway," my boss said. "I don't worry about anyone ever stealing this airplane. There are only a few of these things left; not a whole hell of a lot of people know how to land them. You cut back on her like you do with other planes, you're dead. I would not have to worry about killing the bastard. The plane would do it for me."

I remembered this conversation as we approached the runway. The wheels touched down at sixty MPH. I almost felt safer in the air. I climbed out, wobbled around for a few minutes until I regained my bearings; helped him put the plane away, thanked him for the thrill and went on my way. As I drove towards the job site I couldn't help but wonder why. Why does it seem that there is not much contentment in people; except of course when one is on the edge with adrenaline pumping, or when one is so busy being busy that there is no time to wonder. If only I could be that way all the time. Well here I am, the hammer will take the questions away for today.

Looking back is more painful at times. But in a way it is just more of the same. I am still angry at myself for not questioning the adults in my life. I didn't even think of it. It was all me. My life was in that fool's hands; I did not think I had the right or the ability to take my life into my own. Dangerous stuff. Wrong stuff. Unnecessary.

But it is a done deal. The past is gone and I am still around. I can take responsibility for my life now! If I choose to.

The vines will weaken in time. I can already see that I am getting stronger. Go on, Paul, you're all right.


### STILLNESS

Sailing.
In a stiff and steady breeze.
To much happening to worry.
The wind dies down.
Stranded with self.
Not even a ripple.
Silent.
A heart beat.
A breath.
Rewarding if at peace.
A nightmare when alone.

When the summer arrived, I decided to stop working and just play. That decision was another bad one and only led to more trouble. I needed successes, not idle time. Enough hindsight. I was on my own. I wound up having some good times but never feeling safe or at peace with myself or the past. I was asked to leave the island by the police and left for home, not looking forward to getting grilled by the parents.

They grilled me, then drove me to my next destination, college.

I was full of fear once again. The help that was promised was nonexistent. Anyway my frame of mind was not one to accept help. Why was I asking for special treatment anyway, I wondered. I still thought the problem was just in my head; if I were not so damn lazy, I would be fine. There was no peace to be found. I was trying but I could not find peace for the life of me. The C's and D's and poor effort reports started to trickle in. And with them went my confidence. It was like some sort of social disease; some times, it was unnoticeable; other times you would rather die then pee. The cure was eluding me. In a way, the pain was all I knew. It was what I learned to live with.

"I can do it."

"I can do it."

"Damn it, just leave me alone, I will be okay, I will figure out a way." I made it through the year.

During the first semester of the second year I had an operation on my knee. I thought it was going to be a two day thing. My knee was worse off than the doctor had originally diagnosed. He wound up taking almost all of the cartilage out. I got back to school a week and a half later with a heavily bandaged leg and a pocket full of pain killers.

Getting around in the snow was difficult; trying to catch up was impossible and my sports outlet was history.

I thought, maybe I can't make it. Maybe I should just get the hell out of here before all this kills me. After weeks of debating within, I called my dad.

"Dad, I have to get out of here. It is getting worse, I feel bad and it is building. I am leaving."

"You are always running. Just when you get somewhere where there are people trying and starting to help you, you leave."

"They're not helping me, Dad. I feel horrible and it is getting worse. I have got to get out."

"Well, do not come home."

I left for home the next day anyway. My college days were over forever. I did not need that shit anyway. I would show those bastards. School is a god damn joke.

But can I show myself?

The trees outside my window are changing. I see traces of yellows, reds and browns. Though the leaves are still mostly green. But what is the bright red clinging to the trunk. It's a vine.

At the beginning of fall some vines are noticeable. In the summer they hide themselves well. Everything is in the lush green. But when the days begin to grow shorter and the sun has less time to reach the hidden vine, it looses its chlorophyll before the tree. The tree now is blocking the life from the vine. We can see.

Now all we have to do is get rid of it.

# Chapter 12

## DYING FOR SUCCESS

I was an assistant to the director of research at a private brokerage firm. Within a few months my confidence was building. People liked me at work and I liked the job. I set out to learn as much as I could. It was my last chance, I had to make it.

The job was like learning a new language but it made sense. I moved out of my parents' house and found a place to live closer to the city. A year and a half passed. I was doing well in the eyes of society. I still felt like hell, though. No matter what I did, I could not get the vision of the garbage truck from my unconscious.

I later found an apartment on the upper east side of New York City. I was living two totally separate lives, from night to day, from day to night. I was searching for something outside of me, desperately searching for acceptance that I could believe. By now I did not know exactly what I wanted to fit into. I guess I still just wanted to find some peace of mind.

One cool November morning, the air was like a splash of cold water in my face. I woke abruptly to the brand-new day. The lingering chemicals in my system from the night before were causing havoc in my head. I had grown used to it, though. I had come to believe it was just the way of life. The company limousine met me as usual on the corner of eighty seventh and York. Once I was in the plush surroundings of the car, with a telephone in hand, I could relax. I knew I could hide. It was especially easy to hide in those surroundings, many seemed to be doing the same.

I had extracted a semblance of self-worth out of the job. The whole atmosphere, the excitement, power, and money thrilled me and even seemed to keep me alive. I had something I could hide behind and thought if I did well I would receive the money and power that would make me look and feel better. I could fit. No one could touch me, no one would realize that I really didn't fit in. With the job by day and the drugs by night, I would be all right.

I was not all right, anybody who was not running could have seen that instantly. I felt that there had to be more, much more, but where? The stock market was flying. Every move I made was successful. I just concentrated on making money. Bosses would praise me and it felt good. I felt as if I was sheltered from the powerful storm in my head. But in the back of my mind I still had a feeling of dread, of driving that damn garbage truck. How long could I keep up the running? When would the confusion move back? I was in the eye of a hurricane waiting for the destructive winds to return and destroy what was left of me. I wasn't sure how or why I kept on playing this crazy running game with my life. It was as if the people around me could not see the real me.

I was lost in life and did not want to take responsibility for that fact. Help was not a word in my vocabulary and had not been since the third grade. I thought that people who needed help were weak. I knew that asking for help could be pretty damn painful. I couldn't afford to be vulnerable. If I did ask, who around me could give me a sane answer? I thought if I showed my true vulnerable self I would be eaten for breakfast. I kept on baffling myself and others with my overblown powers of manipulation. Digging my grave of isolation deeper and deeper, I made it so I was alone. Like a ghost in a room full of people, no one could hear or touch me.

That afternoon after the stock market closed, I checked my schedule for the next day and went on my way. Back to oblivion, to alleviate the confusion. Back to my searching.

Thinking of the drugs I had left in my apartment from the night before, I was determined to use them in order to stay away from the cold hell inside of me. Though I had grown used to running, I didn't even remember what it was that I was running from.

When I arrived at my apartment I immediately put on some Rolling Stones, mixed a Mount Gay and tonic and did a couple of lines. I was safe again. The cocaine provided the same feelings of security that the job did, with all the power and control. With the cocaine and booze in my system it did not matter that I was a lost. I took my suit off, put on an old pair of faded jeans and a ratty sweater and headed out to Harlem to "run" with my street friends. I didn't understand how or why I was accepted both on Wall Street and 125th street. Maybe like a ghost I could fit in anywhere. I free-based cocaine with my friends until the wee hours of the morning. Strolling 3rd avenue, I noticed the condensation as the air left my mouth but did not feel the bite in the cold gray November morning in my bones.

Somehow I made it back to my apartment safe, after a long stumbling walk. The drugs started to wear off. I went back out. The night was not over, even though it was four thirty on another cold November morning. This time the cold didn't wake me; it numbed my body, mind, and soul. I went back to Harlem on my own, trying to score some more cocaine. My connection was located in an abandoned, blown out apartment building on 102nd Street. When I walked into the building I noticed that it was much colder in the building than it was outside. It was as cold as I felt only one other time in my life, when I was half dead and in shock after I rolled my Jeep. Being wasted and my ghost-like qualities helped me into the hell. I didn't care. It was a decision made by someone who did not care if he lived.

The building was shattered and so was I. There were addicts passed out all over the stairs. They were sprawled out as if dead. Maybe some of them were.

I was walking into a war zone to join the losing side. I climbed the dilapidated stairs, stepping over the motionless bodies, to the dealers' door. When the dealers opened the door and saw me they immediately slammed me up against the wall and put a rusty knife at my throat.

"Who the hell are you and what the hell are you doing here?"

"I need some more cocaine." I said without fear in my voice or eyes.

"We don't have no drugs man. You must be crazy."

"Yeah, I have been buying coke from you guys, all night, through a friend."

"Who the hell is your friend."

"Willard is the name he runs with." The dealer set me free, and went to talk to his partners. All the while they were looking out the window sweating, in the cold, ready to do anything to survive.

They thought I must have been a cop. No one would be stupid enough to come in here alone. While the dealers conversed, I noticed boxes filled with drugs and automatic weapons in the apartment. I realized that these guys were prepared to shoot up the town if they were pushed. I did not care. I asked for the coke again. The dealers took the last of my cash and gave me some heavily cut cocaine. I went on my way back down to my apartment.

I did not want to let my life pass before my eyes, but it was. It had rained and the dark gray city was shining with the reflection of the lights, something I was incapable of doing. There was no use in crying. I walked on.

A few weeks later I went to Jamaica with a bunch of friends to get away from the city, and to listen to some live reggae. Maybe a change of scenery would help.

The stars where amazing, beautiful in the black sky at night. The days were spent on the beach and snorkeling in the clear, warm water that was multi-colored with life. I swam for hours, trying unsuccessfully to catch these elusive fish in my net, not to keep them, just to see if I could catch one. I never did. The coral reef was an underwater forest teeming and glistening with all sorts of life; some obvious, some not.

One afternoon, joining up with a few buddies, we swam around a bend. I noticed a spot where I could climb out of the ocean onto a towering cliff. It was hard to believe that the cliff once had been under the water itself, soft, growing and colorful. It looked like an awesome place to dive in order to get my blood flowing. It was up in the air if the blood was going to be flowing within or spilling out into the sea. The base of the cliff was sharp under foot yet inviting. I chose my steps carefully while I looked behind me thinking of all the different forms and stages of life, trying desperately to understand. I listened while the others talked of the chances one might have if one chose to dive.

We climbed to about a forty-foot level where there was a suitable ledge. The ledge had some loose stones and I kicked them off, they seemed to float down, then splash. I wanted the best footing possible so I could get a stable jump from the jagged cliff. It was not so much the jagged cliff that I was uncertain about. It was the coral below that looked ominous; I would have to clear it when I dove. It did not look colorful from my forty-foot perch. The coral grew out from the cliff and was under six feet of water. It looked like the coral could have been a foot beneath the surface, though it also could have been thirty feet. I had just come from swimming with it. I knew roughly how deep it was.

"Do you think we can make it?"

"You would need a running start," my friends said.

I thought to myself, it looks good. Scary but doable. All the experiences of diving that I had ran through my mind in a flash. Then everything went into slow motion like when you are having a dream and someone or something is chasing you.

I took some deep breaths. My toes clinched to the edge. The weight of my upper body leaned out over the edge, gravity took me over. I was hesitating at a moment where hesitation could kill. I was on my way, there was no way to change my mind; my toes still clung to the edge. I knew if I didn't spring I would not clear the coral. At the very last moment I pushed out with whatever leverage I had left and all the strength I had.

There were no sounds. There were no more choices to be made. Holding one large breath, I plummeted towards the warm and colorful water that suddenly looked hard and cold. Choosing the swan dive for balance and speed control, I seemingly sailed down. The water was coming fast, my arms came together over head; my fists clenched to break a hole for my body to enter. No pain, no blood, just a powerful rushing sensation ran over me. I fought to get back to the surface. The air felt life-giving as it rushed into my wanting lungs.

My buddies screamed, "Paul, man, you missed the coral by about a foot! You're crazy."

"That was great!" I yelled as I swam to the cliff to climb up and do it again. My body was trembling, I was scared and enjoying it.

As I started climbing I noticed myself being afraid to look back. I thought I was not going to be able to make the climb. My adrenaline had made me dizzy and more aware at the same time. The next time I was going to fall without having a chance to get into position. I would not get the necessary spring. I looked only ahead, breathing erratically as I climbed back up, almost too carefully.

The ledge now felt safe. The climb was horrid, imagining, imagining. After I jumped a few times my friends got tired of watching. They climbed back down and swam back around the bend.

Sitting on the ledge resting and trying to enjoy the incredible scenery, I looked down at myself. My arms were tan and amazingly still strong. I was in a peaceful place, in turmoil, having a hard time enjoying the view. Not much had changed.

Alive and dying but not in nature's way. Yes, I am frightened. I asked myself for the first time, what am I doing? Why do I feel like dying?

At that moment I felt an inner peace. A feeling deep from within said that I did not have to die. There was another way.

Beginning that day, I began working on listening and trying to trust that feeling.

**THE PINE GROVE**

The wind wisps and wistles
Through the pines.
Needles fall,
And make a bed.
Safe and peaceful
Among the squeaking
And swaying.

# Chapter 13

## THE SMILE IS WIDE AND REAL

*A tall and awesome looking evergreen towering over the forest in a remote area way off in the hills said to the smaller pines and hardwood trees, "what the hell are some of you trees doing changing color on me? I am green and I stay green all the year through. Green is the only way to be. You had better get your act together or you will be left out and behind."*

*"But I cannot help it," said a small but strong hardwood. It is just the way I am. It will hurt me if I forget who I am and try to live up to you. Your branches can sway more than mine, can't you see that?"*

*"So what."*

*"When the cold winter winds come whipping in from the north a leafless branch is much easier to hold on to."*

*"Listen to me you little twig. This is a cold hard world that we live in; you had better get used to it now. Be a real tree and be like me."*

*"No. Your way doesn't work for me."*

"What? How the hell can you say no to me? I am seven times your size. I have been around for much longer then you. You fool. You have to listen to me."

"I may be smaller; but I have my own roots that are spread far and run deep. I have to try and listen to them, pine. It is hard enough without having to listen to your babbling. Have you ever tried to listen to your roots?"

"Ummm, I am not sure. I think so. I just do what was done to me."

"That is not being a real tree, pine. Come on take a look around and take a look within. Does the system look like it is working? Did it work for you or are you just resigned to it, afraid to take a risk, afraid to see who you really are?

If you are afraid you're not alone, pine. I am scared out of my tree too at times; but I cannot let that fear stop me from risking and trying to just be with all its peace and uncertainty. We all need to listen to our roots, bark, branches, needles, leaves, cones, acorns, twirly things, sap, wood and local pine. We can work together on this. Maybe we can make it a little bit easier."

"Yeah it would be better."

"We can do what we need to do and respect others enough to give them the chance to do what they need to do."

"Hold on you little twerp. Thinking like you I would have to take a real look at myself. I am not sure that I can do it or if I even want to."

"Give yourself a chance, pine. We can't expect to change everything in a day. Just do what you can for the day. Chill out."

"But I would lose my control."

As the trees were talking they didn't notice that the weather was changing. Change was on its way and who was to say which way the trees would turn? For when change is happening it is so much easier to go along with what you're used to; change is funny that way; it seems even trees have a tough time with ambiguity.

"But I would lose my control," said pine again.

"Control is a tiresome idea, pine. Man, feel this breeze coming up? We are in for it, dude. This early winter storm has caught me with some of my leaves on. I am not sure that I can make it through the night."

"Don't worry too much, I am taking the brunt of it tonight. You will make it, hardwood."

"Thanks, pine. Anyway, this breeze is blowing my leaves off at a decent rate. I am holding fast for now and that is all that I really have anyway. I bet that it is for a reason too. I bet an even stronger blow is coming and by then this blow will have blown my branches leaf-free. Ready for any blow."

"I take back that control bit."

"What do you mean, pine?"

"Well, after listening to you babble about the blows it hit me. I can see that nobody can control the wind, and that it is silly to think that we can. You are right, hardwood. As I look down the hill I can see many stunted, twisted, and vine-ridden trees. There are some risks that need to be made."

"Yeah, let's go for it. It was nice talking with you, pine."

"It is nice to talk with you too, hardwood."

"Lets stay in touch and talk and listen often because even a change to the more natural way is hard."

"All right."

**THERE**

Time to heal.
Time to deal.
Deal with mine.
You deal with yours.
In time.
There for self.
There for others.


So I started trying to listen to my roots and the roots of others on my path; not the roots of the vines that I soon began to see on others and in time was able to see on myself. I began to chop at the vine that was almost as wide as I, twisting to the top.

Where am I now?

I am taking risks. Today I have hope. Today I am damn glad to be alive. Today I love myself and I can give and receive love in return. Today I know that I am not bad. Today I know that I do not have to be perfect. Today I can set out to do whatever I want to do. I can take more risks.

I do not want to say that everything is like a bowl of cherries because that would be bullshit. Taking risks is still a difficult thing, but I am getting better at it with each day that I wake up and try. My job is my life and it is far from over.

Many of the problems I faced and still face today are just part of life. I can deal with that because I have chosen to stand by my side. I have no more need to run, but the option is still there. I must stay on top of the situation; after all, it is my life. I only have now. Fighting the helplessness, I struggled to stay in the reality of what I was accomplishing. I am getting A's and B's; though at times I can still find ways to discount the reality, but I'm not today.

Stay calm. Let the positive roll, it does not need to be explainable. No need to fear. There doesn't have to be an answer. Be aware of the negative, the learned helplessness. You will have a better chance at walking or climbing away from it. I tell myself often.

### GROWTH

The seasons are continually changing.
The clouds roll in then pass.
The trees go with the flow,
And grow.
If they are lucky someone helps them remove vines.

The negative behavior can be obvious or very subtle. It looks to teachers, parents, and self after time like you do not have what it takes to succeed. Looking back, I can see the destructive setup. Only knowing failure, failure was what I came to expect. I made it happen.

The dynamics of the mess are too large too swallow whole, even if you could find the answer in a word. Everyone is different and we all have our own pace. We need to be free to follow the path that we choose. Take what you want for the day and deal the best you can. You might bounce around. You might climb back and forth, from risk to safety, then back again. We have to know that the reachable safer branches are still below and that it is only human to climb around for a time. It is okay to be scared; it is a good sign that you are alive.

It is a choice as long as you know that you have it. Love yourself, you're worth it; you deserve it. Keep on growing and see what happens.

## THE IMPACT ZONE

Through the impact zone.
Energy is ebbing.
The water is cold,
The air is still.
Waves come out of a calm,
Build to potentially crushing proportions.
Too far gone.
Not far enough.
Dive for safety,
Clutching at the sand.
It runs through my fingers.
I lose ground and come up again.
There is one in my face,
It throws me without sufficient breath.
More ground lost.
Survival questioned.
I push on.
There is a lull.
The ocean let me through.
Time to gather thoughts.
Breath.
Energy slowly returns.
Starts to fade.
I can only tread water for so long.
Unreadable.
The slow ache.
My limbs and lungs tell me that it is now or never.
I can see the people on the beach.
I wish I was there.
Warm sand running through my toes.
I watch for a break in the sets.
Rumbling all about.

A tremendous pull, then push.
I'm on my way.
Will I make it all the way back through, the impact zone?
Not enough time for questions.
Time for a breath,
A dive
A grasp.
Turbulence.
Am I sinking or swimming?
A brother comes to the water line.
I see I can make it.

# EPILOGUE

In writing my story I made my learning disability (dyslexia) and the problems that stemmed from trying to fit in to a rigid society when you are different, clearer to myself and my reader.

I needed to do this in order to understand better the ways in which I have reacted and in some cases still react. Primarily because of a consistent bout with learned helplessness and the battle to build self-esteem.

Many are giving themselves up in order to fit in, or dropping out. We all as humans seem to be struggling to find ourselves in a world that needs to put everybody into categories in order to deal with the masses. Is this a fact of life or can something be done in order to help children reach their full potential? I think we have an obligation to the children to help them be the best they can be. I think the problems in the system are obvious. Any attempt to change the system is going to take time and patience; but if the system is not working it needs to be fixed. I can see that I am not alone with these feelings. Anybody with any sort of difference or disability, HUMANS can relate. In writing I helped myself resolve some of the misconceptions. And opened the door to risk, to change.

There are many exceptional people out there that cannot fit in to the society's limited and rigid mold. No one can put a name to what these exceptional people are, so in turn they are rejected, suppressed, cut down and cut off from the mainstream before they have the ability to stand up for themselves. Being different does not have to mean being bad or wrong.

The systems we invent hold many people back from reaching their full potential by setting children up to fail, thus knocking self-esteem. To prevent a person from growing is, in effect, to waste that person. Society, by means of education, family, and peers are all working together with the end result in many cases being that people with a difference develop low self-esteem and "learned helplessness." Thus they never come near reaching their full potential. Some people have told me that that is just the way it is. There has to be a bottom in order for there to be a top. If this is even a tiny bit true and nothing is done about it we as humans are in for it. How can we complain about the woes of society when we are setting them up? That just the way it is crap may be somewhat true but that doesn't make it any less insane.

All of the information I read and wrote about is well known and well documented. However, I had no idea about the magnitude of it all. I know from experience that knowing the realities helps one to change. Learned helplessness written about through a story that people can relate to, allows for better understanding that the life script is wrong and only leads to further helplessness. To better understand this empowers the individual to change.

If everyone understood this process maybe there would be more acceptance of the differences in ourselves and the things we do not understand. Maybe we can learn something and grow more if we do not have to fit everybody and everything into a controllable, nameable place.

It hurts me to know how many people are going down because they are let down by the early education system in this country. The early years are the most important; we have to better help our young people get a confident start in life or we are just asking for the problems in our society to get worse.

The task I have ahead for myself is huge: to leave Mr. Negative on the shelf and stick to the positive. Getting this story out has helped me to get on the road to success.